MO J. ASSELMAN

25 Genuine Moroccan Dishes You Have to Try

An Insider Guide to a Storied Cuisine

One cannot think well, love well, sleep
well, if one has not dined well.

Virginia Woolf

Contents

Author Story

I was born in a northern Moroccan city about ten miles from the azure waters of a Mediterranean beach. The bright white houses are still sprawling over the mountain side, and somewhere near the top, there lies my grandmother's home hamlet.

I grew up in that town and around Morocco, with a heritage of pride, openness, hospitality, and a love for the good life that spans multiple millennia. With the abundance and variety of earth's bounty that our farmers and fishermen were eager to share. In the small market town where I went to primary school, countryfolk often knocked on our door to gift us a bottle of fresh milk, a little basket of eggs, a bunch of carrots, and sometimes a pair of free-range, live chickens. They said their kids were my dad's students.

My mom and grandma made delightful casseroles, hearty soups, and colorful, cheerful salads and oven dishes with such ingredients. They told tales of kings and queens who were so particular about the condiments and seasonings of their foods they just sent off the cooks and made them with their own hands.

It is that spirit that I'd like to share in this book. It is not a cookbook. Yet it is a book that may inspire cooking with tales of flavor and fragrance, spreads, and delicacies with an insider's insight. For those hands-on readers who would like to experiment based on my narrative, I will point to a curated collection of online videos showing one or the other version of each dish.

That open-source content is property of its respective creators, borrowed here gratefully and in fair use. I beg to be forgiven for skipping the translation, but the images will speak for themselves. Wishing you a solid, illuminating and pleasurable read, I would highly appreciate your favorable review on Amazon.

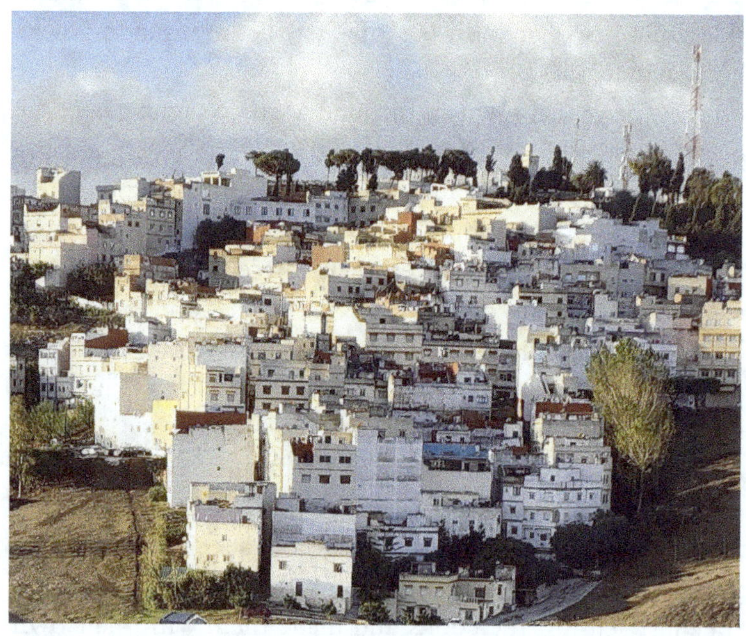

Photo: Mo J. Asselman

History and influences

Moroccan cuisine is a unique and ancient art that stands out among its peers the world over. It is famous for its tasty dishes with a special flavor and aroma. It has a long and varied history. It is said that Hanno, the Carthaginian explorer who sailed along the western coast of Africa in the sixth century BCE, was offered tender mutton in onion, honey and saffron by Moroccan tribesmen he encountered at an ancient trading post.

Today, Moroccan cuisine is widely considered to be the best in the Arab World and Africa, and second only to French cuisine globally. Avenzoar (1094-1162), the Andalusian Arab physician and poet, was commissioned by his caliph to write *the Book of Foodstuffs* (*Kitab Al Aghdiya*), one of the earliest cookbooks in history. At that time, Morocco was a vast kingdom whose rulers controlled territories that stretched from the Senegal River in the south to way beyond present-day Zaragoza, Spain, in the north, and even beyond into southern France.

Morocco's cuisine is a fusion of different flavors, reflecting the diverse cultures and regions that have interacted with the country over time. It combines the ancient practices of the

Imazighen[1] tribes (called barbarians by the Romans), original inhabitants with middle eastern and African influences. A notable European aspect of Moroccan cuisine is the use of fruits, such as quince with meat and apricots with chicken.

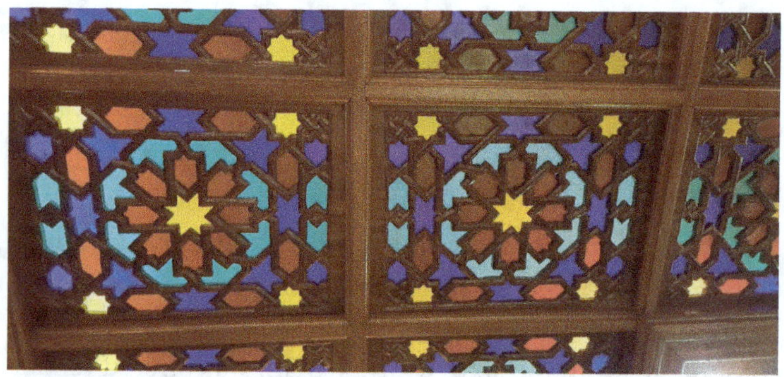

Photo: Mo J. Asselman

---

[1] In the ancient Tamazight national language, spoken by Morocco's First Nations and alive to this day, the word *Imazighen* literally means "Freemen".

Ingredients and spices

A typical Moroccan meal starts with hot and cold salads, followed by the tajine. Bread goes with all dishes, and the next course is often mutton or chicken. Couscous with meat and vegetables comes with buttermilk. Meals usually finish with mint tea. With every bite, scoop, or spoonful, you will experience different eras and civilizations, move between farms, fields, fisheries and their products, and discover cities and villages and their unique identities.

Moroccan dishes are known for the abundance and variety of ingredients used in cooking, as Morocco produces Mediterranean and tropical fruits and vegetables, as well as mutton, poultry, beef, and fish. The widespread but discerning use of herbs and spices is one of the secrets behind the high quality of Moroccan food. These include cinnamon, cumin, saffron, turmeric, ginger, black pepper, paprika, coriander, parsley, thyme, and celery. They are mixed according to fairly strict, long-established rules that Moroccan cooks are reluctant to stray away from.

Most of the food in Morocco is made with different combinations of fresh vegetables. Some of the common ones are carrots, potatoes, tomatoes, turnips (both white and yellow), pumpkin, and onions. Some communities also use lentils or beans (both white and green) in their dishes. Zucchini, eggplant, lettuce, and cucumbers are ingredients for side dishes and salads.

This book is by no means a collection of recipes, nor is it an exhaustive handbook. However, it does offer educated descriptions of a selection of gastronomic marvels. It aims to pique readers' curiosity and kindle their imagination, a significant ingredient in Moroccan cooking. Restaurants around the world take pride in offering these legendary dishes, but the best place to enjoy them is at home.

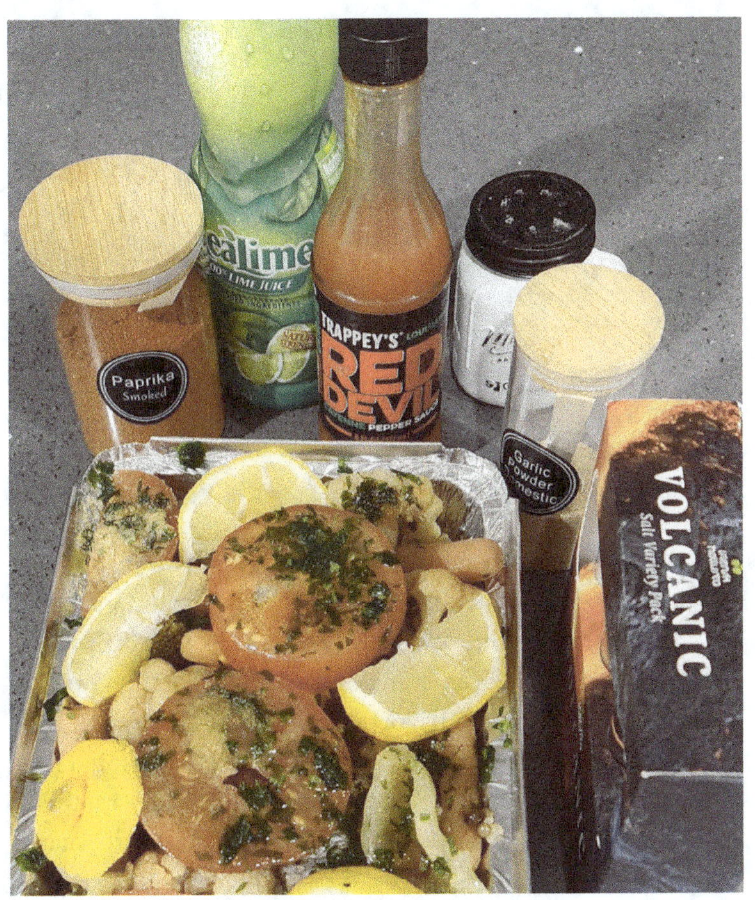

Photo: Mo J. Asselman

Salads and sides

Carrot and pickled lemon

Khizzu Mshermel (seasoned carrots) is a traditional Moroccan salad that is cherished for its unique blend of flavors and textures. The star of this dish is the humble carrot, which is transformed through the cooking process into a tender and flavorful component. The carrots can be cut into any shape or size, adding a touch of personal flair to the dish. Some even prefer to mash the carrots, creating a variant of the dish known as Zaalook dyal Khizzu (carrot mash).

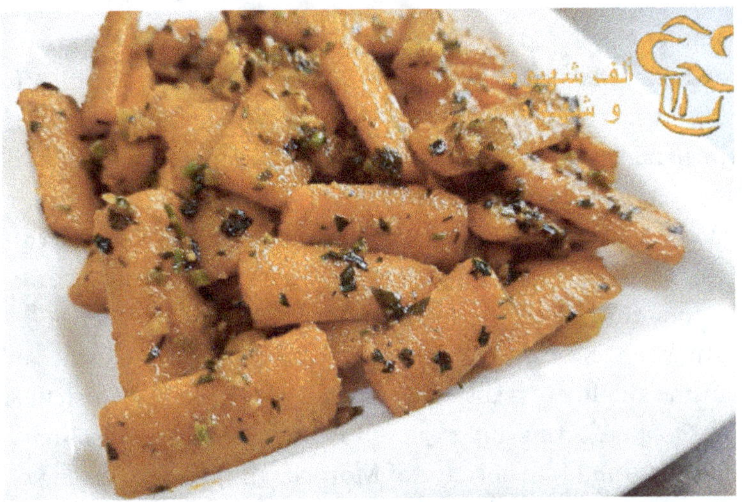

https://www.youtube.com/watch?v=ohrS3D8UUc8 (Chef Siham)

The magic of Khizzu Mshermel lies in the Shermula (seasoning), a traditional Moroccan marinade that infuses the carrots with a burst of flavor. The Shermula is a vibrant blend of fresh herbs, spices, and citrus, creating a balance of flavors that is quintessentially Moroccan. The beauty of Shermula is its versatility - it can be adjusted to suit individual preferences, whether that means more lemon for a tangy kick, extra garlic for a robust flavor, or additional heat for those who enjoy a bit of spice.

Once the carrots have been marinated in the Shermula, they are cooked until tender and then dressed with a drizzle of extra virgin olive oil, a squeeze of fresh lemon juice, and a sprinkle of spices. The result is a dish that is rich in flavor, yet light and refreshing. If the aim is to make a carrot mash, a moderate amount of pickled lemon flesh is added to the Shermula, and lemon peel is used to decorate the servings.

Khizzu Mshermel is not only delicious but also versatile. It can be served as a starter, offering a tantalizing preview of the meal to come, or as a side dish, complementing the main course. This flexibility, combined with its delightful flavor profile, makes Khizzu Mshermel a beloved staple on Moroccan tables, particularly in the city of fez, where it is a family favorite at lunchtime.

In essence, Khizzu Mshermel is a celebration of Moroccan cuisine's ability to transform simple ingredients into a dish that is both comforting and exotic. It is a testament to the culinary creativity and rich heritage of Morocco. Enjoying a serving of Khizzu Mshermel is like taking a bite out of Moroccan culture - a delicious and unforgettable experience.

* * *

Pepper and tomato

The Moroccan salad made with grilled green peppers and fresh tomatoes is known as Tektuka. This traditional dish is a flavorful blend of simple, yet robust ingredients that come together to create a unique culinary experience.

Tektuka starts with green bell peppers, which are charred until tender, adding a smoky depth to the salad. The peppers are then simmered in an aromatic tomato sauce, creating a delightful contrast between the smoky peppers and the tangy tomatoes.

Garlic, parsley, and a variety of spices, including cumin and paprika, are added to the mix, infusing the salad with a bold, spicy kick. The result is a dish that is garlicky, spicy, and lightly smoky.

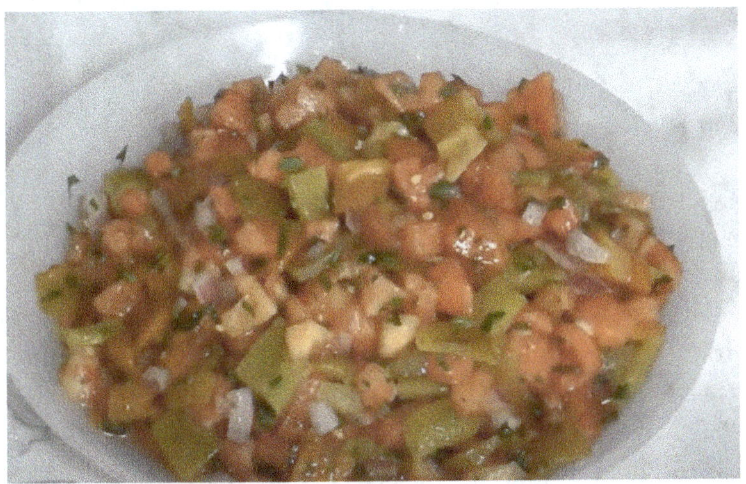

https://www.youtube.com/watch?v=miL2JxwegqA (Ahlam Cuisine)

Tektuka is not just a salad, but a versatile dish that can be served in a variety of ways. It can be enjoyed as a healthy appetizer, a side dish, or even a dip. It's also a common feature in Moroccan gatherings and parties.

What sets Tektuka apart is its texture. It lives in a beautiful middle ground between a salad, a dip, and a stew. The chunky yet brothy consistency, combined with the fresh yet velvety flavors, makes Tektuka a unique and memorable dish.

Tektuka is a dish that showcases how Moroccan cuisine can transform simple ingredients into a meal that is both cozy and exotic. It reflects the culinary inventiveness and diverse heritage of Morocco. Having a portion of Tektuka is like tasting

Moroccan culture - a wonderful and memorable experience.

* * *

Beet and parsley

The Moroccan salad made with steamed or boiled beets is a vibrant and flavorful dish that showcases the natural sweetness and earthy flavor of beets.

The beets, playfully called Barba in Moroccan Arabic, are first prepared by washing them thoroughly under running water. They can then be boiled, steamed, or roasted until tender. The skin of the beets easily slips off once they are cooked. In Morocco, beets are often sold by the bunch, which can make it difficult to select uniform-sized beetroot for even cooking. Cutting the beets into same-sized pieces can help with that, and smaller pieces also mean less cooking time and therefore better preservation of the health benefits.

Once the beets are cooked and the skin has been removed, they can be sliced, cubed, or coarsely chopped. The beets are then tossed in a light vinaigrette. For the best flavor, it is recommended to allow at least an hour for chilling and marinating. The salad can even be made a day or two in advance. Today, creative Moroccan cooks have revisited this summer treat by adding a teaspoonful of mayonnaise to each serving.

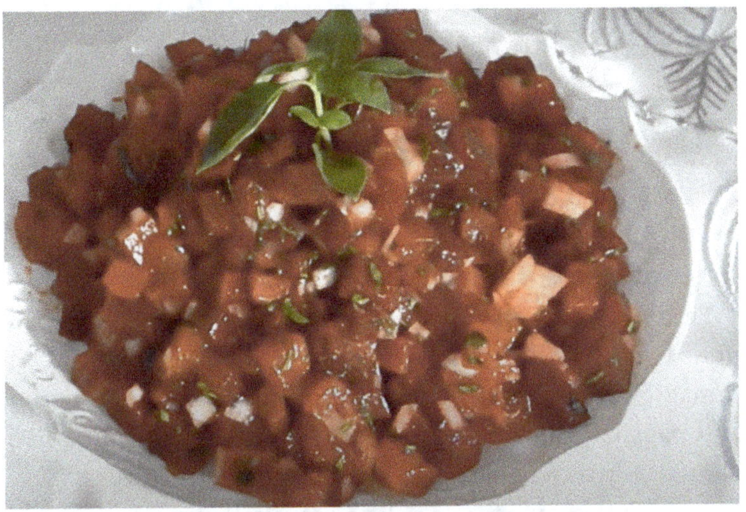

https://www.youtube.com/watch?v=LBPUgsmh4eU (Ahlam Cuisine)

This beet salad is not only delicious but also incredibly healthy. Beets are a super-food with antioxidant, anti-inflammatory, and detoxification benefits. They're also high in vitamin c and fiber and rich in minerals such as potassium and manganese[2].

The Moroccan beet salad is a favorite in many homes. It's a simple, yet delicious dish that adds a beautiful pop of color to any meal. Whether served as a side dish or a main course, this Moroccan beet salad is sure to impress with its fresh flavors and healthful ingredients.

* * *

---

[2]   Medical News Today, https://www.medicalnewstoday.com/articles/27743 2, accessed April 2024.

Eggplant and tomato

Mashed eggplant and tomato, or Zaalook, is a popular Moroccan dish that is often served as a dip or side dish. It's primarily made from eggplant and tomatoes, seasoned with a variety of spices and herbs.

The eggplant is first peeled and diced, then boiled or roasted until tender. The cooked eggplant is then combined with tomatoes, garlic, and a blend of warm spices including cumin and paprika. This mixture is cooked down to a puree-like consistency, although some prefer a chunkier texture.

Zaalook is known for its rich and savory flavor, which comes from the combination of earthy eggplant, tangy tomatoes, and aromatic spices. It can be served hot or cold and is traditionally enjoyed with Moroccan bread.

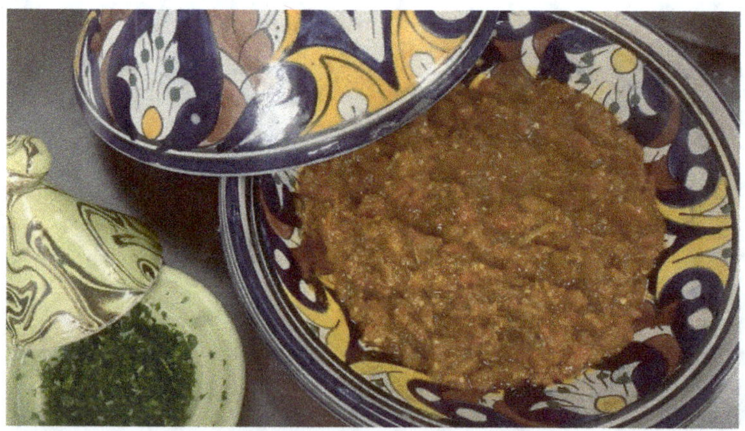

https://www.youtube.com/watch?v=OIgiqb9loAs (Chef Nadia)

This dish is not only delicious but also versatile. It can be used as a spread on bread, as a dip for vegetables, or as a side dish to complement other Moroccan dishes. Its robust flavor and comforting texture make it a favorite in many Moroccan homes.

In essence, Zaalook is a celebration of the simplicity and depth of flavors in Moroccan cuisine. It showcases how humble ingredients like eggplant and tomatoes can be transformed into a dish that is both comforting and full of flavor.

* * *

Lettuce and cucumber

The Moroccan salad made with lettuce and cucumber is a refreshing and light dish, perfect for a hot summer day or as a palate cleanser during a rich meal. The salad is simple, consisting of crisp lettuce and fresh cucumbers, but it's the dressing that truly brings it to life. The dressing is typically a blend of olive oil, lemon juice, salt, and pepper, whisked together until emulsified. This simple vinaigrette adds a tangy brightness that complements the cool crispness of the lettuce and cucumber.

Some variations of the salad may also include sliced tomatoes, red onions, and fresh herbs like coriander or parsley for added flavor and color. This salad is a testament to the Moroccan culinary philosophy of using fresh, local ingredients and enhancing their natural flavors with simple, yet effective seasonings. It's a versatile dish that can be served as a starter, side dish, or even a light main course.

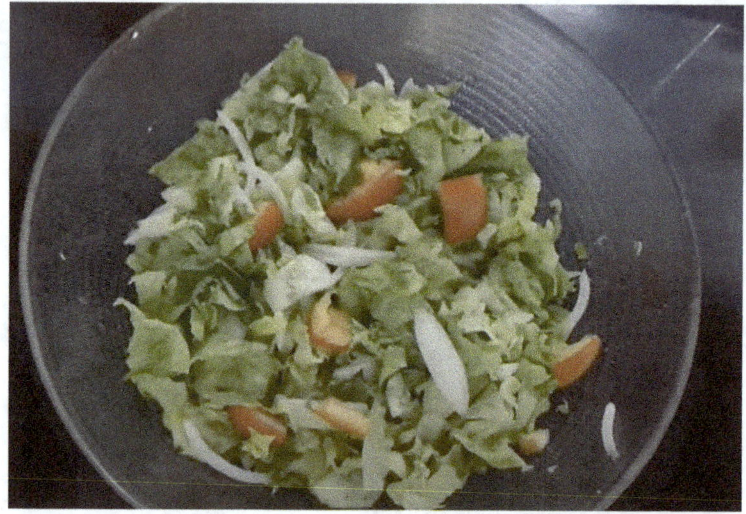

https://www.youtube.com/watch?v=HbVOJAG0GkE (Wasafati Cuisine)

Cucumbers are a healthy choice due to their high-water content, which contributes to overall hydration and digestion. They are rich in vitamins, minerals, and antioxidants[3]. The high potassium content can be part of a diet to lower blood pressure, and they are also rich in vitamin k, which plays an essential role in bone health.

Lettuces, like romaine, green and red leaf, and butter lettuce, promote good health. They are nutritious vegetables that contain antioxidants, fiber, folate, omega-3 fats, calcium, and other vitamins and minerals. Green leafy lettuces also contain the antioxidant vitamin k, which may decrease the blood-

---

[3] Health.com, https://www.health.com/nutrition/health-benefits-cucumbers, accessed April 2024.

thinning effect of warfarin[4].

Lettuce is a healthy high water content vegetable. The nutrient content of lettuce varies depending on the type eaten. Most lettuces are good sources of vitamins k and a. These minerals support bone and vision health. Lettuce contains fiber which keeps the digestion process running smoothly.

____

4 Lettuce Info, https://lettuceinfo.org/lettuce-nutrition/, accessed April 2024.

Soups

Hareera

Hareera is a traditional Moroccan soup that is rich in flavor and hearty in texture. It is primarily made from tomatoes, lentils, and chickpeas, and is robustly seasoned with ginger, pepper, and a variety of fresh herbs. Cinnamon is optional, and raging debates ensue when the question of its pertinence as an ingredient of Hareera is raised among Moroccan chefs.

The preparation of Hareera involves cooking the lentils and chickpeas until tender, then adding them to a fragrant tomato-based broth. Some variations of Hareera also include meat, such as mutton, beef, or chicken. The soup is typically thickened with either broken vermicelli pasta or rice.

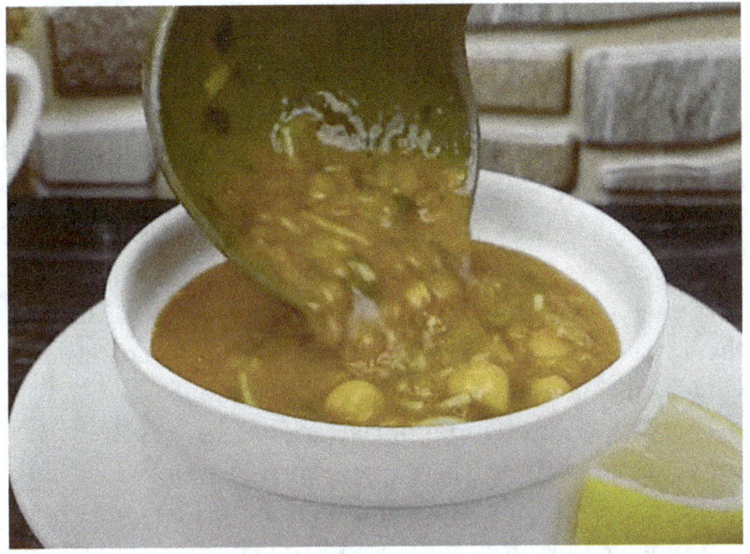

https://www.youtube.com/watch?v=4wdfnQdYOa4 (Jannat Kitchen)

Hareera is famously associated with the holy month of Ramadan, when it's often served to break the fast. However, it's also enjoyed year-round in Morocco and other parts of North Africa. The name Hareera, derived from the Arabic word for silk (hareer), makes reference to the soup's velvety texture.

This soup is not only delicious but also nutritious. The lentils and chickpeas provide a good source of protein and fiber, while the tomatoes contribute vitamins and antioxidants[5]. Whether served as a starter or a main course, Hareera is a comforting and satisfying dish that truly embodies the flavors of Moroccan cuisine.

---

[5] Healthline, https://www.healthline.com/nutrition/chickpeas-nutrition-benefits, accessed April 2024.

Hareera, like many traditional dishes, has regional variations that reflect the diverse culinary traditions within Morocco. The recipe and ingredients can vary depending on the region. For example, some parts of Morocco make Hareera with rice or vermicelli noodles, while others may use mutton instead of beef. Even the spices and vegetables can vary, especially as they have been adapted to different parts of the world. The recipe presented in fez, known as Fassi Hareera , is often considered the "real" Hareera . Fassi cuisine, renowned for its nobility and elitism, distinguishes itself by its sophistication.

There are also variations of Hareera that have evolved over time. For instance, Khatifa is a porridge cooked in milk and accompanied by salted butter. Khazira is boiled bran accompanied by diced meat, and Rista consists of pieces of boiled meat, chickpeas, lentils, and hand-rolled vermicelli.

* * *

Bissara

Bissara is a traditional Moroccan soup that is both hearty and nutritious. It's primarily made from either dried split peas or fava beans[6], or sometimes a combination of both.

The preparation of Bissara involves boiling the peas or beans until they are tender. Garlic is added during this process, infusing the soup with its robust flavor. Once the peas or beans

---

[6] Healthline, https://www.healthline.com/nutrition/fava-beans, accessed April 2024.

are cooked, they are blended to create a smooth, creamy texture.

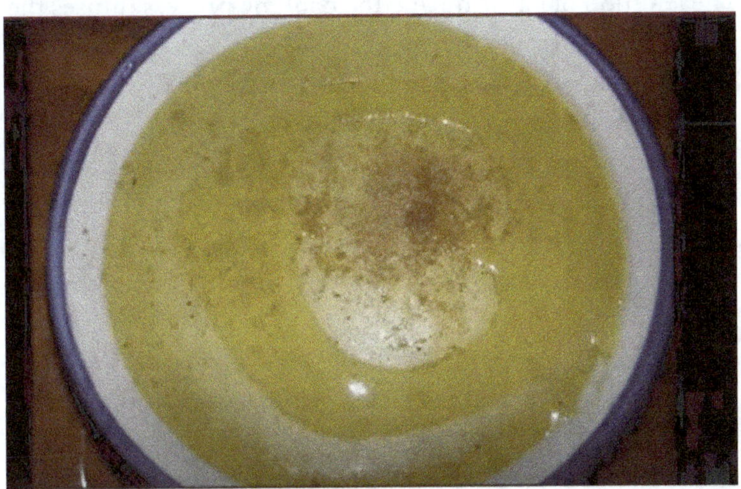

https://www.youtube.com/watch?v=dzu6-cfXc3c (Chef Oum Riad)

Olive oil is a key ingredient in Bissara, adding a rich depth of flavor and a silky mouthfeel. The soup is seasoned with a variety of spices, including cumin and paprika, which give it a warm, earthy taste. A lot of connoisseurs throw in a dash of fresh lemon juice, but never more than half a teaspoonful.

Bissara is not just a soup, but a versatile dish that can be served in a variety of ways. It can be enjoyed as a dip with crusty bread or served as a soup with a drizzle of olive oil and a sprinkle of cumin and cayenne pepper.

This humble dish is a testament to the simplicity and depth of flavors in Moroccan cuisine. It showcases how simple ingredients like peas, beans, garlic, and olive oil can be transformed into a comforting and satisfying meal.

Bissara is a favorite during the winter months. Its warmth

and heartiness make it an ideal comfort food for cold evenings. The addition of garlic during the cooking process infuses the soup with a warming touch.

What makes Bissara a perfect winter fix remedy is its nutritional value. It's very healthy, easy to prepare, and filling all at the same time. The peas or beans provide a good source of protein and fiber, making Bissara a substantial meal that can keep you feeling full and energized on cold days.

Moreover, Bissara is often enjoyed at any time of the day in Morocco, even for breakfast. It's also one of those dishes that allow you to socialize over the same bowl of yumminess. The soup is typically served with a generous drizzle of olive oil, a sprinkle of cumin and paprika, and fresh chopped onions are a must in the northern areas of the country. Other regions include hot sauce as an essential component. These additions not only enhance the flavor but also add to the soup's comforting qualities.

* * *

Mixed veggies

Moroccan cuisine is renowned for its rich and diverse range of soups, many of which feature a medley of vegetables. These soups are not only delicious but also nutritious, offering a hearty and comforting meal that showcases the fresh produce and aromatic spices characteristic of Moroccan cooking.

One such soup is the Moroccan pureed vegetable soup. This soup is popular in many parts of Morocco and uses a variety of vegetables, traditionally used in the famed Moroccan couscous, such as carrots, cabbage, pumpkin, and turnips. Running the cooked ingredients through a hand-operated vegetable mill produces a mouth-watering, grainy texture. In modern times, electric food processors, mostly blenders, are used to create light, smoothie-like bowls of comforting nourishment. The ingredients can be adjusted based on personal preference and what vegetables are on hand.

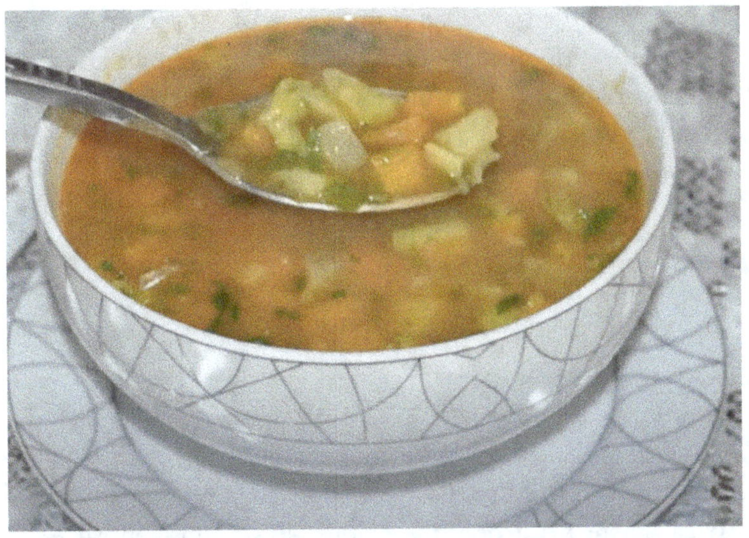

https://www.youtube.com/watch?v=XT93-b_duGU (Chef Safae Oum Arwa)

Another example is called Shorba, a ubiquitous soup in Moroccan cuisine that comes in many different versions. Made with a mishmash of vegetables, this soup can be cooked with any type of protein, including chicken, beef, or mutton.

A modern Moroccan spiced vegetable soup with couscous is another variant that includes salty Kalamata olives, tender artichoke hearts, protein-packed chickpeas, and canned tomatoes served with a scoop of couscous. All the ingredients come together to create a soup full of flavors and textures.

These soups are typically seasoned with a variety of spices, including turmeric, and paprika or saffron, which add depth and complexity to the flavors. They can be enjoyed as a starter, a main course, or even a light snack.

In essence, the mixed vegetable soups of Moroccan cuisine are a celebration of the country's abundant produce and rich culinary traditions. They offer a delicious and nutritious way to enjoy a variety of vegetables, making them a beloved staple in Moroccan homes and beyond.

* * *

Vermicelli

Moroccan vermicelli soup is a traditional dish enjoyed by North Africa, Eastern Europe, the Middle East, and Central Asia, with each country having its own unique variation. It is often confused with Shorba, but in Moroccan cuisine, vermicelli soup often includes chicken and diced carrots and onions.

One popular version of Moroccan vermicelli soup is a clear type of soup, typically with chicken and vermicelli noodles in it. It's a different take on the chicken noodle soup model, being a little more robust and more colorful. Some recipes make the broth in the soup, while others use pre-made vegetable broth.

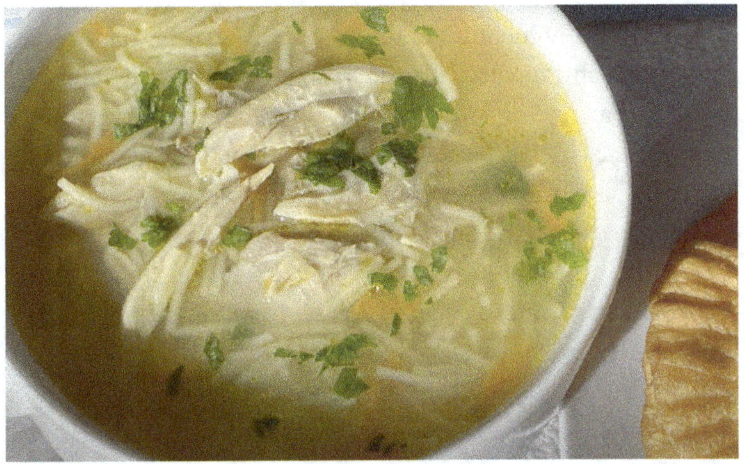

https://www.youtube.com/watch?v=atRO7-VPda0 (Zeina Cuisine)

Moroccan vermicelli soup may have mutton or chicken, chick-peas or carrots, sometimes both. It is tomato and broth-based and uses lighter aromatics, such as a bouquet of fresh herbs like parsley and cilantro, lemon juice, and ginger. There aren't typically any heavy spices such as those used in Moroccan Hareera .

Vermicelli soup and classic chicken soup are both comforting, hearty soups, but they differ in their ingredients, preparation, and cultural origins. Vermicelli soup is seasoned with a variety of spices, including turmeric, and paprika, which add depth and complexity to the flavors. Some versions of vermicelli soup also include celery, and tomatoes. The soup is often enjoyed during Ramadan, to alternate with Hareera , but it's also a staple in Moroccan homes year-round.

On the other hand, classic chicken soup, often associated with American and European cuisines, is a simple and comforting dish. It typically includes chicken, carrots, celery, and onions, cooked in a chicken broth. Some recipes also include herbs like thyme or parsley for added flavor. Unlike Moroccan vermicelli soup, classic chicken soup usually doesn't include legumes like chickpeas, and the spices used are often less varied.

In terms of preparation, both soups involve simmering the ingredients until they are tender. However, revisited versions of Moroccan vermicelli soup often involve the additional step of blending the broth and vegetables to create a smooth, creamy texture, before adding the vermicelli and returning the mix to the stove, on low to medium, to simmer for ten to fifteen minutes.

* * *

Lentils

Moroccan lentil soup is a hearty and nutritious dish that is a staple in Moroccan cuisine. It's primarily made from lentils, often combined with other ingredients such as tomatoes, onions, and a variety of spices. The soup is known for its rich, earthy flavor, which is enhanced by the addition of spices like cumin, turmeric, and paprika. Some purists advise against cumin and paprika, insisting that authentic lentil soup should be made with black pepper and saffron. Some also point out that this dish is actually not a soup, and that the water content must be reduced to the least possible, giving it a hardier, less fluid consistency.

The preparation of Moroccan lentil soup involves boiling

the lentils until they are tender, then adding them to a fragrant broth. Some versions of the soup also include vegetables like carrots, celery, and even cubed pumpkin, as well as proteins like chicken or beef. The soup is typically served with a squeeze of fresh lemon juice and a sprinkle of fresh herbs, adding a bright, fresh element that balances the hearty flavors of the lentils. Purists again say extra virgin olive oil and hot sauce are the true finishing touches, with meat and poultry being big no-noes.

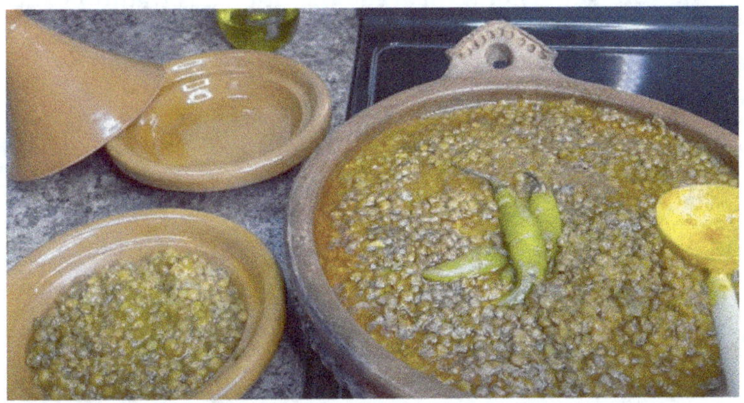

https://www.youtube.com/watch?v=7_i5yraRjuc (Chef Nadia)

In addition to being delicious, Moroccan lentil soup is also incredibly nutritious. Lentils are a great source of protein and fiber[7], making this soup a satisfying and healthy choice. Whether enjoyed as a warming lunch on a cold day, or as a comforting dinner at the end of a long one, Moroccan lentil soup is a beloved dish that truly embodies the flavors and

---

7   Medical News Today, https://www.medicalnewstoday.com/articles/29763
    8, accessed April 2024.

traditions of Moroccan cuisine.

Speaking of lentils as a versatile ingredient in Moroccan cuisine, one popular dish is the Moroccan lentil salad. This salad is infused with fragrant Moroccan spices, crunchy celery, toasted almonds, dried apricots, and orange zest. The lentils are cooked until tender, then tossed with the other ingredients and a flavorful dressing. This salad is not only delicious but also highly nutritious, making it a perfect choice for a healthy lunch or dinner. Purists call this salad an aberration, but chefs of the younger generation argue that it blends tradition and innovation perfectly.

but I digress!

Tajines

Chicken, olives, and pickled lemon

Moroccan chicken tajine with olives and preserved lemons is a classic dish that is rich in flavor and history. The dish is named after the traditional clay or ceramic pot it's cooked in, which has a unique cone-shaped lid that helps to retain moisture and enhance the flavors of the food.

The preparation of this dish begins with marinating the chicken in a mixture of garlic, saffron, ground ginger, paprika, turmeric, and black pepper. For the marinade, it's always the longer, the better, but by no means less than a couple hours. The marinated chicken is then browned and set aside to make room for a pile of thinly sliced onions, which are sauteed until golden brown. The chicken is then nestled back into the pan, along with slices of preserved lemons and olives. A bit of chicken stock and lemon juice is added, and the dish is cooked over low heat until the chicken is tender, and the flavors have melded together.

Preserved (or pickled) lemons are a key ingredient in this dish, adding a unique tangy flavor that can't be replicated with fresh lemons. The olives, both Kalamata and cracked green olives, add a salty, briny flavor that complements the other ingredients. The dish is typically served with some sauce, lemons, and olives over the chicken. Fresh, whole-wheat bread or Italian bread, liberally dipped in the sauce, are an essential part of the meal.

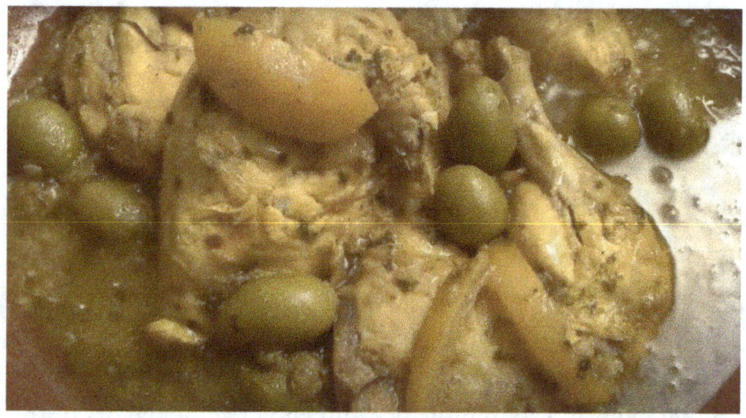

https://www.youtube.com/watch?v=dc26WoK3mrw (Anonymous Moroccan in Canada)

This dish is a testament to the depth and complexity of Moroccan cuisine. The combination of savory chicken, tangy preserved lemons, and salty olives creates a balance of flavors that is both comforting and exotic. Whether enjoyed in a mountainside cafe in Morocco or in the comfort of your own home, Moroccan chicken tajine with olives and preserved lemons offers a culinary experience that is sure to please.

Moroccan chicken tajine with olives and preserved lemons is a classic that has several variations, reflecting the rich culinary diversity of Moroccan cuisine. One variation involves the addition of different vegetables, such as potatoes, onions, and tomatoes. The vegetables are coated in the same marinade as the chicken and arranged around the chicken in the tajine. This version of the dish offers a more robust flavor profile and a greater variety of textures.

Another variation of the dish includes different types of olives. While the classic recipe calls for green olives, some versions use Kalamata olives or one of the many types of olives available on the Moroccan market. These olives have a variety of sizes, colors, and flavors, which can add a unique twist to the dish every time. A third variation involves the use of different spices. While the traditional recipe calls for a blend of spices including coriander, turmeric, and cayenne pepper, some versions may include additional spices or adjust the quantities to suit individual preferences.

* * *

Beef and prunes!

Moroccan Osso Bucco with dried prunes or apricots is a delightful fusion of Italian and Moroccan cuisines. The dish is traditionally made with veal shanks, but beef can also be used. The meat is braised in a sweet and savory sauce, enriched with a blend of warm Moroccan spices.

The key ingredients of this dish include veal shanks or beef, onions, garlic, ginger, white pepper, beef or veal stock, dried apricots, prunes, and a variety of spices such as harissa, paprika, cayenne pepper, turmeric, cinnamon, and saffron. The dish is cooked slowly in a pot, a pressure cooker, or in the oven, allowing the flavors to meld together and the meat to become tender.

There are several variations of this dish. One variation involves the addition of different vegetables, such as potatoes or bell peppers. Another variation includes different types of dried fruits, such as dates or figs, instead of apricots and prunes. Some recipes may also include different spices or adjust the quantities to suit individual preferences. Regardless of the variation, Moroccan Osso Bucco with dried prunes or apricots is a flavorful and satisfying dish that showcases the rich culinary traditions of Morocco.

Adding sesame seeds to Moroccan Osso Bucco with dried prunes or apricots can enhance the dish in several ways. The sesame seeds are often toasted before being added to the dish. Toasting the seeds brings out their natural oils and intensifies their nutty flavor. This can add a new layer of complexity to the dish, complementing the sweetness of the prunes or apricots and the savory flavors of the beef.

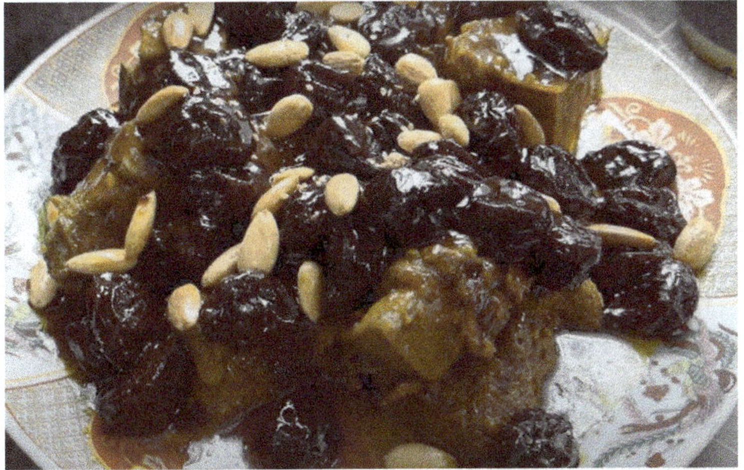

https://www.youtube.com/watch?v=jvyCM-kGh5U (Chef Majda Berrada)

In addition to flavor, sesame seeds also add a delightful crunch to the dish. This contrast in texture can make the dish more interesting and enjoyable to eat. Halved, hard-boiled eggs are sometimes arranged around the meat for a stunning visual effect.

Moreover, sesame seeds are highly nutritious. They are a good source of fiber and plant-based protein, and they are rich in various vitamins and minerals, including b vitamins, vitamin e, magnesium, zinc, and calcium[8]. Therefore, adding sesame seeds to the dish not only enhances its flavor and texture but also boosts its nutritional value.

In some variations of the dish, sesame seeds are used as a garnish, sprinkled on top of the dish just before serving. This

---

[8] National Library of Medecine, https://www.ncbi.nlm.nih.gov/pmc/articles /PMC9573514/, accessed April 2024.

not only adds a nice crunch and flavor but also makes the dish visually appealing.

***

Mutton and veggies

Moroccan mutton tajine with mixed vegetables is a traditional dish that showcases the rich flavors and culinary techniques of Moroccan cuisine. The dish is named after the tajine, a clay or ceramic pot with a cone-shaped lid used to cook this dish and numerous others, which helps retain moisture and enhance the flavors. In large, popular restaurants nowadays, the ingredients are cooked separately in pressure cookers but served in tajine pans as individual or family portions.

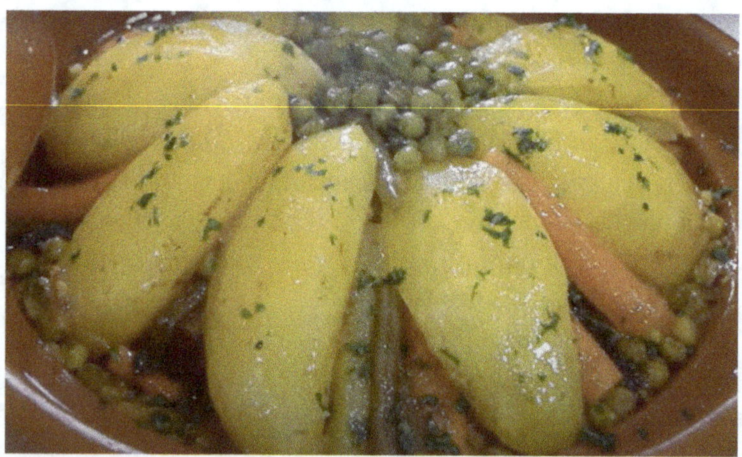

https://www.youtube.com/watch?v=vCc4Rh6wPm8 (Chef Nadia)

The preparation of this dish involves marinating the mutton in a mixture of spices, including turmeric, paprika, and others. The marinated mutton is then slow cooked with a variety of vegetables such as carrots, onions, and potatoes. Some versions also include other vegetables like bell peppers or green beans. The slow cooking process, often over a charcoal fire, allows the flavors to meld together and the mutton to become tender.

There are several variations of this dish. Some recipes include different types of vegetables or adjust the quantities of spices to suit individual preferences. Other variations might include different types of dried fruits or nuts for added flavor and texture. Regardless of the variation, Moroccan mutton tajine with mixed vegetables is a flavorful and satisfying dish that truly embodies the flavors and traditions of Moroccan cuisine.

Creating this storied Moroccan dish begins with the mutton. The meat is lovingly coated in a paste made from a blend of spices, including turmeric, and ginger, combined with garlic and olive oil. This marinated mutton is then introduced to a hot pressure cooker or a Dutch oven, where it's browned to perfection on all sides.

While the mutton rests, thinly sliced onions take its place in the pot, sauteing until they turn a beautiful golden brown. The mutton then returns to the pot, nestling among the onions. A fragrant broth is created with the addition of vegetable stock, providing a bath for the mutton to cook in.

The pot then welcomes the vegetables, which can range from artichoke and fresh peas to cauliflower and sweet potato. The whole dish is now slow-cooked, either in a pressure cooker or in an oven preheated to 300 degrees F. This slow cooking process, whether it's over a charcoal fire or in a modern kitchen, allows the flavors to meld together and the mutton to become tender.

The final touch to this dish is the addition of dried fruits. Depending on the variation, this could be prunes, apricots, dates, or figs. These dried fruits add a touch of sweetness that balances the savory flavors of the mutton and vegetables. It is worth mentioning that many versions include green cracked olives, pitted olives or Kalamata.

The result is a flavorful and satisfying, long-celebrated dish that truly embodies the flavors and traditions of Moroccan cuisine. Whether it's prepared in a traditional tajine over a charcoal fire or in a modern kitchen using a pressure cooker or oven, the essence of the dish remains the same - a celebration of Moroccan flavors and culinary techniques.

* * *

Meatballs and eggs in tomato

The Moroccan dish made with meatballs, tomatoes, and eggs is known as Tajine Kefta Kwary, the Moroccan meatball tajine. This popular dish features meatballs, known as Kefta Kwary or Kefta Mkewra, cooked in a zesty, homemade tomato sauce. The meatballs are typically made from ground beef and are seasoned with a variety of herbs and spices including paprika, cumin, salt, pepper, onion, parsley, and cilantro. Some recipes also include garlic, turmeric, and even ginger.

The meatballs are cooked in a tomato sauce, which is often spiced with cayenne pepper or whole chili pepper for a bit of heat. Many cooks like to present the meatball tajine with eggs poached directly in the sauce, but this addition is optional. The eggs, when broken, create a creamy sauce that adds richness to the dish.

This dish is traditionally cooked in a tajine, a clay or ceramic cooking vessel, but it can also be prepared in a deep skillet. The slow cooking process allows the flavors to meld together and the meatballs to become tender. Moroccan tradition is to gather round the tajine and eat communally from the dish, using pieces of Moroccan bread to scoop up the meatballs and sauce.

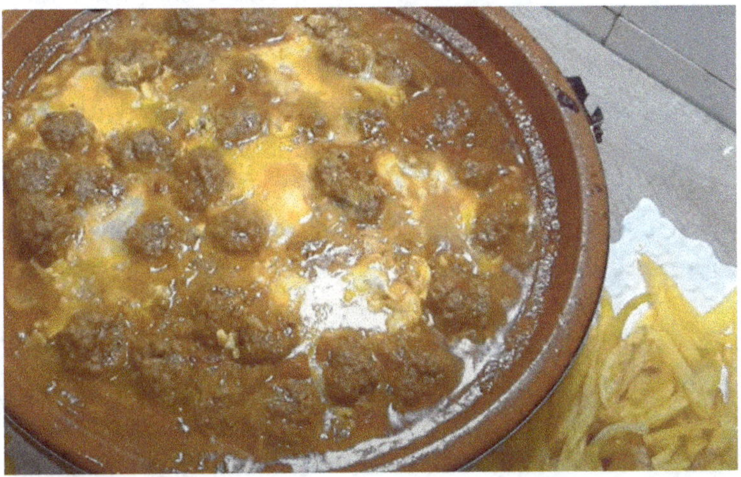

https://www.youtube.com/watch?v=fyQcMdtMM6M (Chef Oum Faty)

There are several variations of this dish. Some recipes include different types of vegetables or adjust the quantities of spices to suit individual preferences. Other variations might replace the eggs with potatoes for added flavor and texture. Regardless of the variation, the meatball tajine is a flavorful and satisfying dish that truly embodies the flavors and traditions of Moroccan cuisine. Some new-wave chefs recommend serving a side of French fries with the tajine, or even throwing a liberal amount of your favorite grated cheese. Purists would object vehemently.

Speaking of potatoes, some chefs offer a wildly different but equally delightful variation known as Batata bel Kefta, which features meatballs and potatoes. The spices remain the same to a large extent, although the focus shifts to the herbs. It must be pointed out that this is a rather recent variation, typically prepared in a stainless-steel pot or a pressure cooker, carefully taking timing into account.

The potatoes are peeled, washed, and diced into half-inch cubes. The ground beef is lightly salted and mixed with olive oil, black pepper, cayenne pepper, a little cumin, garlic powder, fresh chopped coriander, and paprika. The potato cubes are rolled in mix of pepper, parsley, cilantro, freshly crushed garlic, with either turmeric or paprika, never both. Many adventurous chefs swap the herbs mentioned here for rosemary, thyme, basil, chives, dill, bay leaves, fennel, lemongrass, and even oregano.

The spiced and seasoned meatballs and potatoes are then slow cooked in not more than a cup of water and a ¼ cup of olive oil. The potatoes add a hearty element that complements the savory meatballs. With perfect timing, they also tend to melt partially, producing a delightful, unctuous dip that fresh bread just loves.

* * *

Seasoned sea bream

Fish tajines are a staple in Moroccan cuisine, offering a delightful blend of flavors and textures. The dish is traditionally prepared with a firm, thick fish such as meager, sea bass, or sea bream. Indeed, with the country's near 2,000-mile coastline spanning the Mediterranean Sea in the north and the Atlantic Ocean in the west, Moroccan men who cook maintain that the fish species hardly matters. It's all about the Shermula. One will concede that women chefs are more particular, even picky, but nonetheless masterfully creative.

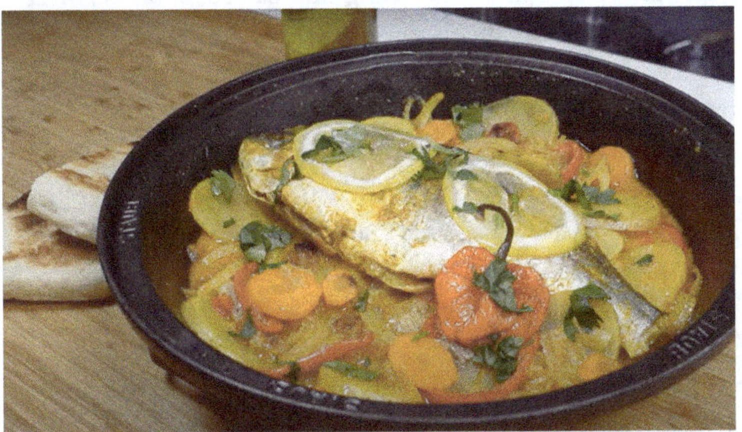

https://www.youtube.com/watch?v=Ep2fPhuiEds (Food Is Love)

The fish is marinated in the zesty herb and spice mixture, then layered with vegetables like potatoes, carrots, tomatoes, and green peppers in a tajine for slow braising. The conical lid of the ubiquitous earthenware pot creates a seal that allows the steam to ascend and then condense, subsequently returning into the container. This acts as a natural and continuous basting of the food being cooked.

Seasoned sea bream tajine is a particular variant of the Moroccan fish tajine. The sea bream is marinated in a mixture of spices, garlic, and olive oil. The marinated fish is then nestled into the pot, along with slices of preserved lemons and olives. A bit of chicken stock and lemon juice is added, and the dish is cooked over low heat until the fish is tender, and the flavors have melded together.

Whether it's prepared in a traditional tajine over a charcoal fire or in a modern kitchen using a stove and a deep skillet, Moroccan fish tajines, including the sea bream tajine, offer a culinary experience that is sure to please. The sea bream, a firm, thick fish, is an excellent choice for this dish thanks to its rich flavor and texture.

The Shermula brings the often-underrated sea bream to a high level of sophistication by penetrating the fish, enhancing its natural taste. The marinated fish can also be cooked with thinly sliced onions sauteed to a beautiful golden brown. Sometimes, the fish is surrounded with slices of preserved lemons and olives.

One variation of sea bream tajine involves adding vegetables such as zucchini and bell peppers. The vegetables are sliced finely and fully covered with Shermula. The dish is then transferred to the oven and cooked until the vegetables are half cooked and start to soften. The fish fillets are then added on top of the vegetables and the dish is placed back in the oven for 8 to 10 minutes depending on the thickness of the fish. This turns the "lowly" sea bream into a feast of delight and sophistication.

Couscous and Co.

Seven veggies

Moroccan couscous with seven vegetables, also known as Couscous Bidawi, is a traditional dish that originated in the countryside around Casablanca, Morocco's sprawling metropolis locally called Dar El-Beida, literally, The White House. Couscous is widely considered the ultimate comfort food to enjoy with family and friends. It is often washed down with large glasses of fresh, chilled buttermilk.

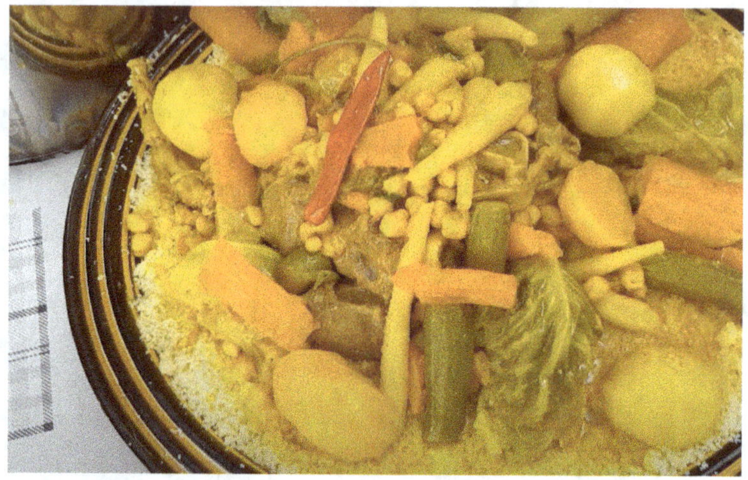

https://www.youtube.com/watch?v=Rsdmqa-yqV4 (Moroccan Flavor)

The dish typically includes mutton, beef, or chicken stewed with assorted vegetables, then served atop a mound of light, fluffy steamed couscous. A rich broth seasoned with ginger, pepper, and turmeric is poured over all or offered on the side. The vegetables used in this dish can vary, but the common ones include onions, carrots, pumpkin, zucchini, turnips, cabbage, and chickpeas. However, the number seven in the dish's name is more of a guideline; more or fewer vegetables may end up in a particular cook's version of couscous with seven vegetables.

The couscous is traditionally steamed while the meat and vegetables are stewed. The dish is often garnished with Tfaya, a caramelized onion and raisin topping. It's worth noting that you can omit the meat for a vegetarian version. The dish can also be made gluten-free by using a corn semolina, instead of the usual durum wheat or barley version. In place of fresh meat or poultry, dried meats such as Gueddid can be used.

In the southwestern cities of Safi and Essaouira, big fish such as tuna and swordfish replace the meat and poultry. In this case, fist-size pieces of fish are first cooked in the rich broth made with olive oil and a mixture resembling Shermula, the cook's imagination being the only constraint. To avoid overcooking the fish or causing it to break up into unseemly bits, it is set aside while the choice of veggies boil in the sauce and the semolina is prepared. Unlike the typical Couscous Bidawi and its countless variations, it is strongly advised not to serve buttermilk with fish couscous. Try fruit juice, sugar-free soda, or plain old mint tea instead.

* * *

Sweet cinnamon

Couscous Tfaya is a traditional Moroccan dish that features couscous and a sweet and spicy caramelized onion and raisin garnish known as Tfaya. The star spice here is cinnamon, more than in any other version. The dish is typically served with meat or poultry but generally prepared without vegetables. Pints of cold buttermilk are again called for.

The Tfaya garnish is a key component of this dish. It's made by cooking onions and raisins from a pale stage to a caramelization stage with honey or sugar. In addition to the cinnamon, Tfaya is seasoned with aromatic spices such as ginger and saffron. Most versions of couscous Tfaya also include chickpeas.

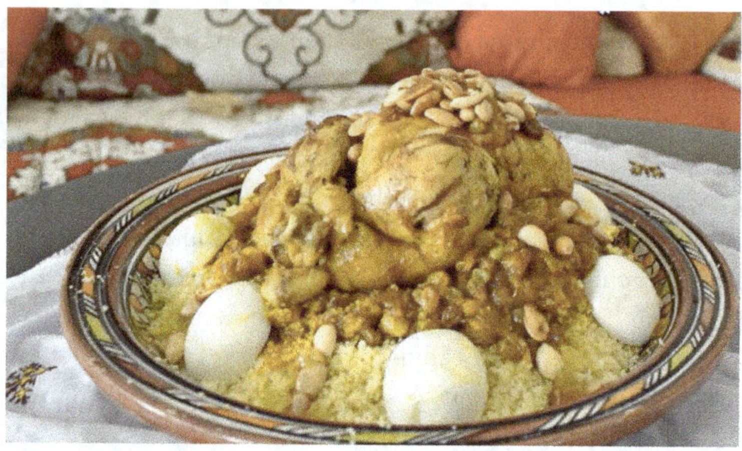

https://www.youtube.com/watch?v=AV2ZUKiWB90 (Chef Halima Filali)

The couscous in this dish is ideally steamed over the simmering meat. You can use either chicken or mutton in this recipe. The ingredients call for the special, fragrant spice blend known as Ras El-Hanoot, literally "top of the shop", a mix of the top 10-15 spices in refined spice stores, often with the store owner's exclusive touch. If you can't find it, you can substitute a few whole cloves and a pinch of nutmeg.

Fried almonds are a common, additional garnish and can be made ahead of time. They are quickly boiled or soaked in piping hot water, peeled, and deep-fried until golden brown. They are then placed atop the Tfaya on a bed of couscous.

There are also vegan versions of this dish. For example, one recipe replaces the meat with chickpeas and cranberries. Once again, some purists are adamant that free-range chicken is the only acceptable protein-source to be covered with the noble Tfaya, to which some attribute medicinal properties.

* * *

Shredded flatbread and chicken

In the heart of Morocco, where tradition weaves through the streets like the intoxicating scents of spices, there lies a dish that is the very essence of Moroccan culture: Rfissa. This cherished meal is more than just sustenance; it is a story on a platter, a narrative of flavors passed down through generations.

Rfissa is akin to couscous in that both involve steaming the grain-based ingredient. Imagine a dish where the warmth of shredded, puffed flatbread would compete with the tender embrace of thinly cubed corn pancakes. This is the canvas upon which Rfissa is painted. The main characters in this culinary tale are none other than succulent chicken and hearty lentils, both brought to life with a symphony of spices that dance upon the palate.

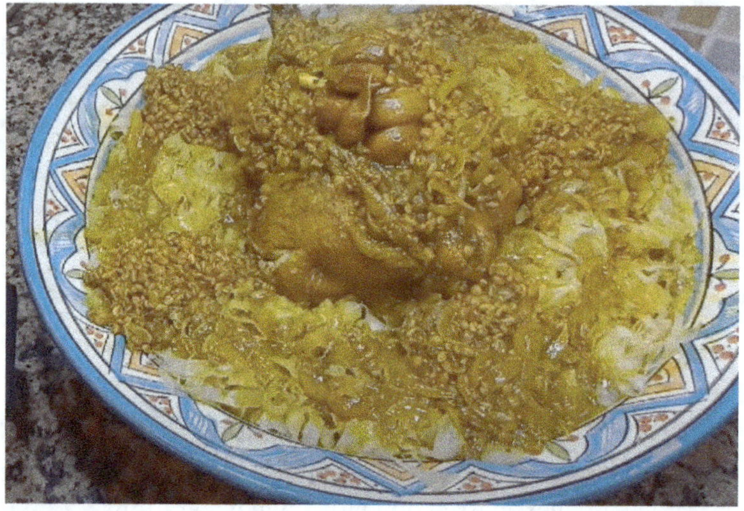

https://www.youtube.com/watch?v=j-MRDMjEiLM (Chef Halima Filali)

The preparation of Rfissa is a ritual in itself. The chicken, bathed in a marinade of onions, olive oil, and a medley of spices including ginger, turmeric, and the fabled Ras El-Hanoot, is cooked to perfection over a gentle flame. Lentils, cilantro, parsley, and a pinch of saffron join the ensemble, simmering together in harmony. Meanwhile, Msemmen, the Moroccan flatbread, is torn into delicate pieces, each layer steamed to softness, ready to soak up the flavors of the stew.

Rfissa's roots run deep, tracing back to Treed, a dish that itself harks back to Thareed, an ancient Arab creation. Yet, Rfissa stands alone, a variation that has found its own place in the hearts of those who savor it.

Nutritionally, Rfissa is a treasure trove, offering a bounty of protein from the chicken and lentils, along with an array of vitamins and minerals to nourish the body.

But Rfissa's significance transcends its ingredients. It is a dish of celebration, often gracing tables during life's special moments. It holds a special place for new mothers, for whom the fenugreek seeds[9] are said to offer restorative properties. Gathered around the generous platter, people come together, each person partaking from their side, sharing not just a meal, but a moment in time.

And what do the purists say? To many, Rfissa is the epitome of Moroccan comfort food. A dish that warms the soul, comforts the heart, and delights the senses, perfect for any and all occasions. It is, in every sense, a dish that tells the story of a people and their enduring love for the flavors of home.

* * *

Drumsticks and wings under vermicelli

Would the mention of drumsticks and wings under vermicelli transport you to the sun-kissed streets of Tangiers, where flavors dance and memories linger? If yes, the whispering aromas of Seffa Medfoona will be your guide.

In the heart of this cosmopolitan northern city, where the air hums with secrets and the sun paints the walls in warmth, there is a culinary treasure known as Seffa Medfoona. Its name, like a whispered promise, evokes visions of saffron-scented alleys

---

9   WebMD, https://www.webmd.com/diet/health-benefits-of-fenugreek, accessed April 2024.

and bustling marketplaces.

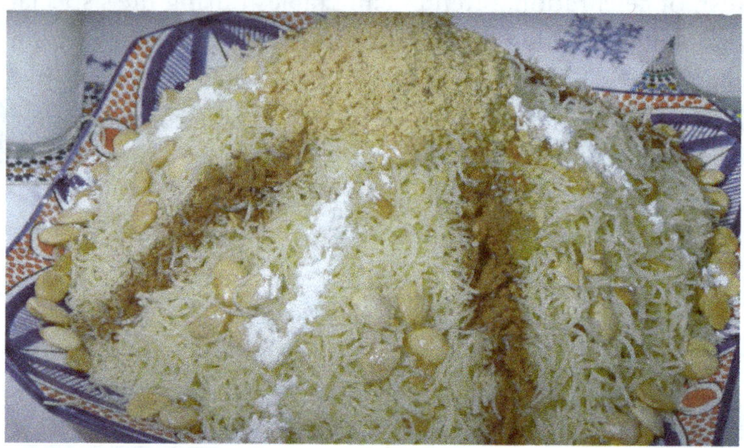

https://www.youtube.com/watch?v=rqsf2m_93lk (Amina Cuisine)

Picture this: a cool courtyard in the summer, where a mosaic-tiled table awaits. The air is thick with anticipation as the hostess, her hands adorned with henna and silver bangles, unveils a platter. There it lies—a mound of steamed broken vermicelli, delicate as spun gold. The grains, like tiny sunbeams, cradle a hidden treasure.

The unassuming looks of the dish are misleading, for within this golden nest lies the heart of Seffa Medfoona —a choice of tender, succulent chicken drumsticks and wings, selected from the youngest birds, marinated in a saffron-infused elixir. The poultry delicacies are buried within the vermicelli, waiting to be discovered. Each strand carries the memory of green fields and ancient grains.

But Seffa Medfoona is no ordinary dish. It wears a dual cloak—a sweet and savory embrace. As if the sun and moon conspired, the dish is garnished with raisins, their plumpness echoing distant vineyards. A hint of cinnamon dances across the surface, while ground almonds add a nutty whisper. And then, like a final benediction, a gentle snowfall of powdered sugar settles upon the creation.

In Casablanca, where the sea meets the fruitful countryside, a different tale unfolds. Here, Seffa Medfoona takes on a new guise—a meat-free version, served as a follow-up course. It tiptoes after the main dish, a harmonious encore. The couscous, now the star of the celebration, weaves its fine grains into a symphony of flavors.

Venture farther—to Meknes and fez—and you'll encounter Seffa Touba. This vegetarian rendition, like a whispered prayer, omits nuts. The couscous, sprinkled with orange flower water, becomes a canvas for simplicity. It's a light dinner, shared under the moon's watchful eye, alongside a comforting glass of cold or warm milk.

As you savor each bite, know that this dish transcends mere sustenance. It carries stories—the laughter of grandmothers, the clinking of silverware, the warmth of shared moments. And yes, it provides 413 calories per portion, but those numbers fade against the tapestry of taste.

* * *

Exclusive! Couscous with zucchini and milk

(A Guarded Family Secret!)

Most Moroccan couscous recipes include zucchini. However, one would be hard-pressed to obtain a specific recipe that uses only zucchini and milk. Of course, recipes can often be adapted to suit individual preferences. But among the hundreds of Moroccan families I know personally, including my in-laws, none have ever heard of couscous with zucchini and milk only. Consequently, I cannot link to a video, but with the AI-generated image below, you'll get the idea.

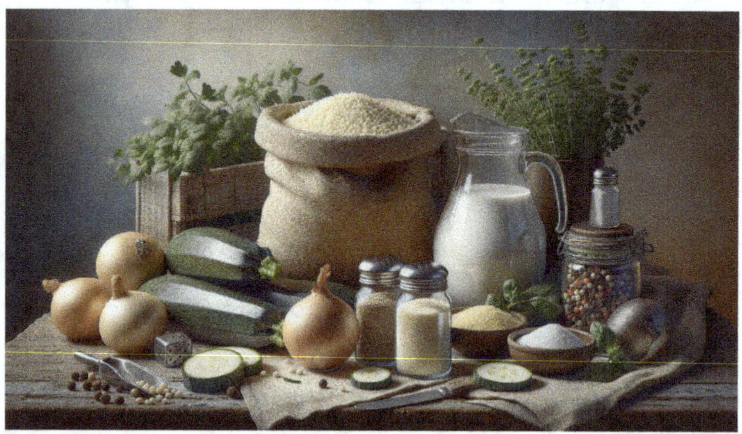

Image: Mo J. Asselman, DALL-E 3. No video found.

The fact is, I suspect this is a creation by my own mom, or maybe my grandma. During the fall months when we lived in a tiny agricultural village where my dad taught school, they used to make us a simple couscous dish with zucchini and a milk-based sauce. It was really no big deal, ingredient and spice-wise.

They would steam couscous in the age-old, typical way, in a colander-type top part of the specific pot used for steaming, known in French as a *couscousier* or *couscoussière*.

In the lower part of the pot, in about two liters of water, they would boil no more than a chopped up, sauteed half onion with salt and pepper. They added in five *courgettes*, or zucchini, each sliced longitudinally and cut up in three sections, making up exactly 30 pieces. I have no idea why that was the number but there were never any leftovers.

When the couscous was steamed and fluffed three or four times, it was mixed with a little olive oil, sometimes butter. The pot remained on the stove to reduce the sauce by evaporation, until it barely just covered the zucchini. It ended up looking a refreshing, energetic light green, to which a liter of milk and a dash of oregano were added and brought to boil. Depending on the zucchini quality, I surmise, Mom occasionally threw in a sugar cube or two.

In a huge, heavy earthenware plate, Mom or Grandma would then top the couscous mound with steaming hot zucchini and shower it with the boiled mixture of milk and cooking juices. The hardest part of the meal was having to wait, tablespoon in hand, for this secret charm to cool down before digging in. Afterwards, it was usually bedtime stories and sweet dreams.

Grill, oven, and steam

Roast mutton shoulder

Across the Moroccan lush and bountiful heartland, at the foot of the rugged Atlas Mountains, an antique dish transcends mere sustenance. Roast mutton shoulder, generically called L'ham M'hammar because it can be crafted with several types of meat, is indeed a famed sensory voyage.

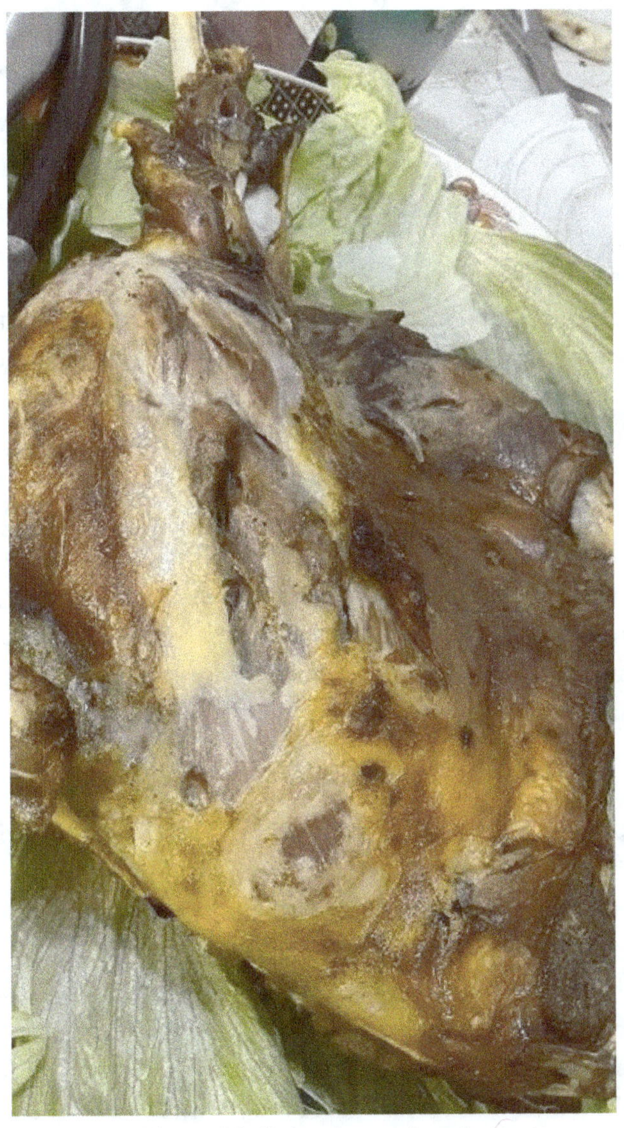

Photo: Mo J. Asselman. See also https://www.youtube.com/watch?v=NNWxkJf4Ty4 (Chef Oum Fawzie)

In many a bustling Moroccan kitchen, the air thick with the fragrance of spices, seasoned cooks have long made L'ham M'hammar for momentous occasions, such as Eid El Ad'ha, special guests, or just at the end of profitable market days. The star of this gastronomic symphony is none other than a mutton shoulder, tender and yielding.

The ritual begins with a marinade—a dance of flavors. Sliced onions, their pungency softened by olive oil, mingle with salt, pepper, ginger, and turmeric. The pièce de résistance is once again the expertly selected Ras El-Hanoot, the spice blend that whispers of distant caravans and ancient trade routes. This aromatic concoction envelops the mutton, infusing it with promises of warmth and comfort.

Next comes slow-cooking — an art form in its own right. The mutton nestles into a clay pot, its fibers surrendering to the gentle heat. Hours pass, and the kitchen becomes a sanctuary of anticipation. The meat absorbs the essence of the spices, turning a deep, golden to burnished red. It's as if the sun itself has seeped into every fiber.

And then, the grand finale—the roasting. The oven door creaks open, revealing the mutton, its edges crisped and inviting. The aroma escapes, filling the room. The family gathers, their eyes alight with appetite. L'ham M'hammar graces the table—a dish that transcends mere sustenance.

But this dish is not confined to Eid El Ad'ha, the festival of sacrifice, locally called Eid El Kebeer, literally the Greater Holiday, Eid El Fitr being the Minor Holiday, or Eid Es Seghir, which marks the end of the month of Ramadan. No, roast mutton shoulder spills beyond those sacred days. At weddings, birth celebrations, and intimate family gatherings, L'ham M'hammar takes center stage. It unites generations, bridging the gap between tradition and modernity.

The taste just defies words. Each bite unravels stories—the nomads who traversed deserts, the traders who bartered for spices, and the artisans who shaped the clay pots. But it's not just about flavor; it's about nourishment. The mutton, tender and yielding, offers sustenance—a promise of strength and resilience.

So, dear reader, if you chance upon L'ham M'hammar, do not hesitate. Take that first bite, close your eyes, and let Morocco embrace you. For within its folds lies not just a dish, but a legacy—a testament to the artistry practiced in Moroccan kitchens and the love that binds families around them.

* * *

Mutton skewers

Let me take you back to the bustling streets of a sunny Moroccan town, where the air is rich with the aroma of spices and the sizzle of grilling meat. Picture this: Kebab or Qotban, the beloved skewered delights that dance over the coals, a symphony of mutton cubes paired with just the right amount of fat to make each bite a juicy, flavorful escapade.

Imagine the days leading up to Eid El Ad'ha, the anticipation palpable in every home, as families prepare to grill these succulent morsels. The secret? A marinade that's a love letter to the palate, infused with garlic, olive oil, and a squeeze of lemon juice, then serenaded with coriander, parsley, mint, pepper, and a sprinkle of cayenne powder for good measure.

For a good two days, these cubes of potential sit patiently, soaking up every note of flavor. Then, with the care of an artist, they're threaded onto skewers, ready to meet the grill. A few minutes each side, and voilà! A feast fit for royalty, or just a gathering of friends and family under the Moroccan sky.

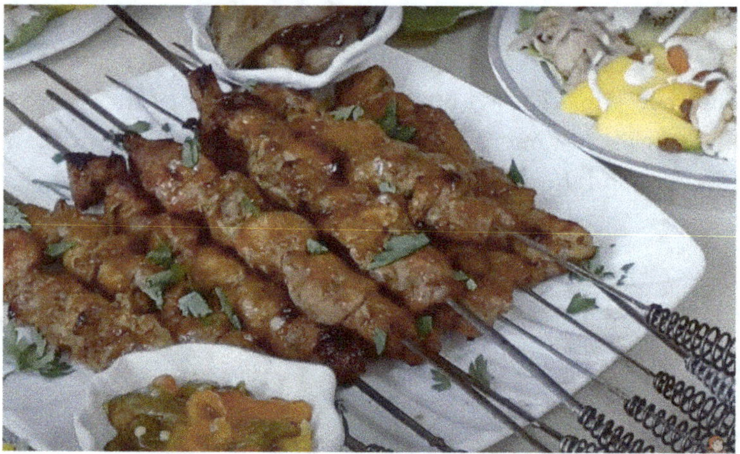

https://www.youtube.com/watch?v=OeHktYy4e84 (Nany Delights)

And let's not forget the variations! Whether it's mutton or beef, the addition of fat is not just tradition, it's a culinary hug that ensures each kebab is as tender as a first love. While the fat may not be everyone's cup of tea, its role in this gastronomic ballet is undeniable. And speaking of tea, it is an absolute must with this particular dish. It has to accompany the grilled meat and fresh bread throughout the meal, while a second pot is brewing on the last coals where the skewers were brought to life.

Variations include liver or white fish cubes, prepared in much the same manner. Moroccan skewers, with their tapestry of textures and flavors, therefore stand shoulder to shoulder with the greats of French and Italian fare. The journey begins with a rub of sweet paprika, ginger, and the mysterious Ras El-Hanoot, setting the stage for a culinary experience that's nothing short of magical.

* * *

Ground beef on coals

The dish we are looking at now is reminiscent of the Moroccan Kefta Kebab or Qotban Kefta, a delightful blend of ground beef or mutton, seasoned with a medley of spices and herbs, then shaped into patties or skewers. These kebabs are traditionally grilled over coals, which imparts a smoky flavor that's utterly irresistible.

As the kebabs sizzle on the grill, they're often accompanied by slices of sweet onions and ripe tomatoes, which caramelize and soften, adding a touch of sweetness and juiciness to the meal. The combination of the savory meat with the charred vegetables creates a harmonious balance of flavors that's both comforting and indulgent.

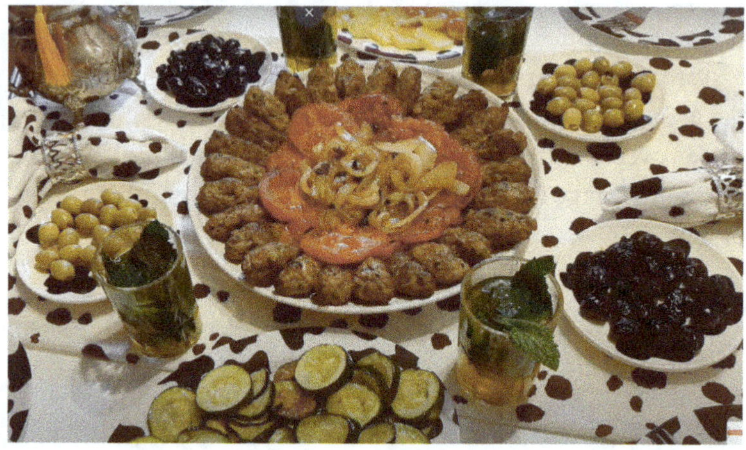

https://www.youtube.com/watch?v=jB-lCy87yGU (Nadifatrigo)

In Morocco, such dishes are not just about the food; they're an experience, a celebration of culture and tradition that brings people together. Whether it's a family gathering or a festive occasion, the act of grilling and sharing Kefta kebabs is a cherished ritual that evokes a sense of nostalgia and communal joy.

The spices that grace the Moroccan Kefta kebab are not just ingredients; they are the storytellers of a rich culinary heritage. Each pinch of cumin and paprika whispers tales of bustling souks and vibrant landscapes, while minced onion, coriander, and parsley add layers of fresh, herbaceous notes to the narrative. Optional yet impactful, the warmth of turmeric and the kick of cayenne pepper join the chorus, with mint leaves offering a refreshing finale that lingers on the palate. These spices, each with their own distinct voice, come together in harmony to create a melody that sings of Morocco's soulful food symphony.

As for the accompaniments, imagine sipping on a glass of Moroccan mint tea, affectionately known as 'Moroccan whiskey', its sweetness perfectly balancing the robust flavors of the kebabs. Or perhaps a smoothie, blending tropical fruits like pineapple, mango, and avocado, to provide a sweet, tangy counterpoint to the savory meat. On the side, a simple yet elegant Moroccan carrot salad or a small plate of Zaalook, the eggplant salad, could grace the table, adding color and a medley of textures to the feast. These sides and drinks don't just complement the kebabs; they elevate the entire dining experience to an art form, a celebration of flavors that's quintessentially Moroccan.

* * *

Steamed mutton

In the heart of Moroccan cuisine lies a dish that is simplicity and tradition wrapped in one: the steamed mutton shoulder and ribs. This dish, often prepared during the festive days following Eid El Ad'ha, is a testament to the time-honored methods of Moroccan cooking. The mutton, chosen for its rich flavor and tenderness, is steamed for several hours until it reaches a state of buttery perfection, effortlessly falling off the bone.

The preparation begins with large cuts of mutton, generously seasoned with salt and pepper, and sometimes a touch of saffron for an extra layer of flavor. These pieces are then lovingly coated with soft unsalted butter or a traditional fermented butter, which adds a depth of flavor that is uniquely Moroccan. The meat is placed in a steamer or couscousier, the special pot used for steaming couscous, and left to cook slowly, allowing the steam to work its magic. A modern pressure cooker with a suitable-size strainer or colander are used nowadays to save time.

As the mutton cooks, the aromas that fill the kitchen are a prelude to the feast to come. The steam carries with it the essence of the herbs and spices, infusing the meat with the flavors of parsley, cilantro, and coriander. This bouquet of herbs not only seasons the mutton but also creates an aromatic environment that is a hallmark of Moroccan gastronomy.

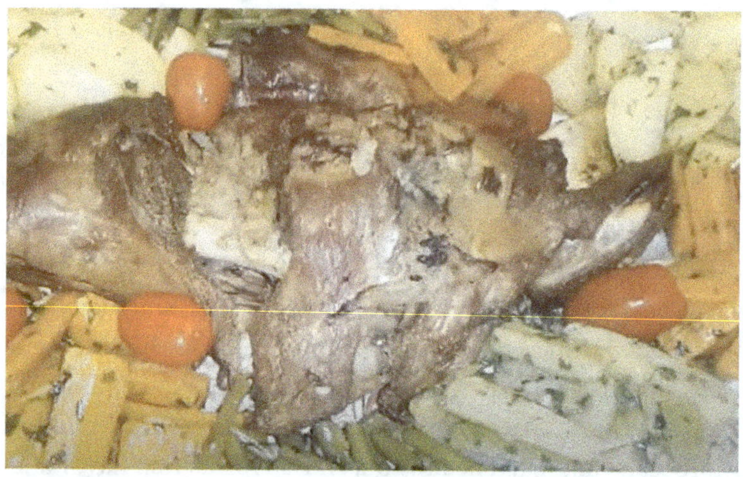

https://www.youtube.com/watch?v=ngp4-oedrBU (Atbak Ch'hiwat Bladi)

Accompanying the mutton are often vegetables such as carrots, potatoes, and onions, which are added to the steamer in the latter stages of cooking. These vegetables soak up the flavors of the mutton and the herbs, becoming tender and flavorful themselves. They are not just sides but integral components of the dish, contributing their textures and tastes to create a well-rounded meal.

To serve, the steamed mutton is presented with cumin and salt on the side for dipping, a simple yet essential pairing that enhances the natural flavors of the meat. This dish is not about complexity; it's about celebrating the ingredients' inherent qualities and the joy of sharing a meal that has been prepared with patience and love. It's a dish that brings people together, around a table filled with warmth, laughter, and the shared experience of a meal that is deeply rooted in Moroccan culture.

* * *

Grilled sardines

A platter of Moroccan-style oven-grilled sardines, a dish that captures the essence of the sea with a symphony of flavors, both bold and delicate, is often the central attraction of summer days. These sardines, glistening with olive oil, are adorned with slivers of garlic, a medley of herbs, and a vibrant array of bell peppers and tomatoes, creating a mosaic of colors and tastes that are quintessentially Moroccan.

The sardines are first prepared with meticulous care, cleaned, gutted and de-boned, leaving behind only the promise of their rich, omega-3 laden flesh[10]. They are then marinated in a blend of traditional spices and herbs, including the likes of cumin, coriander, and a hint of chili for warmth. This marinade not only infuses the fish with flavor but also tenderizes them, ensuring that each bite is succulent and full of zest.

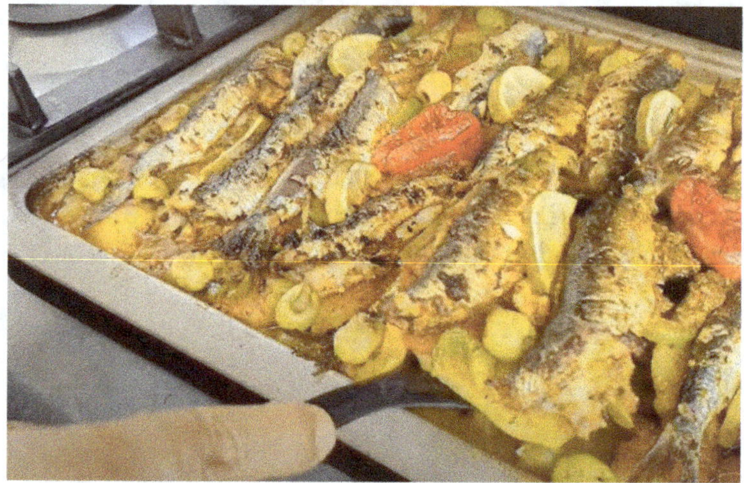

https://www.youtube.com/watch?v=TO31xJ-eMSA (Chef Souad)

As they're placed in the oven, the sardines are set in pairs and layered with thin slices of bell peppers and tomatoes, which roast and sweeten, releasing their juices to mingle with the fish. The garlic caramelizes at the edges, turning golden and fragrant, its aroma mingling with the herbs to create an intoxicating scent that beckons one to the table.

The cooking process is a gentle one, with the heat of the oven

---

[10] WebMD, https://www.webmd.com/diet/health-benefits-sardines, accessed April 2024.

enveloping the sardines in a warm embrace, allowing them to cook to perfection. The result is a platter of sardines that are crispy on the outside, yet tender and moist on the inside, with the vegetables transformed into a soft, sweet bed that complements the fish's natural flavors.

To serve, this dish is often accompanied by a fresh, crusty bread to sop up the flavorful juices, and perhaps a side of Tektuka, the Moroccan salad made with roasted bell peppers stewed in an aromatic tomato sauce. The combination of the oven-grilled sardines with these sides creates a meal that is not just nourishing but also a celebration of Moroccan culinary traditions, a feast for the senses that is both humble and grand in its simplicity.

* * *

* * *

Conclusion

Mo J. Asselman recounts his upbringing in a northern Moroccan city near the Mediterranean coast. The town, a tableau of white houses sprawling across the mountainside, holds memories of the author's grandmother's home hamlet. Growing up in Morocco, the author experienced a rich heritage of pride, hospitality, and a love for life. Farmers and fishermen generously shared the bounty of Earth and Sea, and countryfolk often gifted fresh milk, eggs, carrots, and even live chickens. The author's mother and grandmother prepared delightful dishes, emphasizing the importance of condiments and seasonings. Although not a cookbook, the author's work aims to inspire cooking through flavorful tales and an insider's perspective, accompanied by curated online videos.

The author highlights Moroccan cuisine as a unique, ancestral art, renowned for its flavorful dishes and distinctive aroma. Its rich history dates back to encounters with Carthaginian explorer Hanno, who enjoyed tender mutton seasoned with onion, honey, and saffron. Presently, Moroccan cuisine is celebrated globally, ranking second only to French cuisine. Avenzoar, an Andalusian Arab physician and poet, authored the early cookbook, called authoritatively *The Book of Foodstuffs.*

Morocco's culinary heritage blends Imazighen (Berber) traditions with Middle Eastern and African influences, featuring the creative use of fruits like quince and apricots in savory dishes.

The essence of Moroccan cuisine lies in its diverse and flavorful dishes. A typical Moroccan meal begins with hot and cold salads, followed by tajine. Bread accompanies every dish, and mutton or chicken often follows. Couscous with meat and vegetables is served alongside buttermilk. Meals conclude with refreshing mint tea. Each bite transports you through different eras and civilizations, revealing unique identities. Moroccan cuisine boasts an array of ingredients, including Mediterranean and tropical fruits, mutton, poultry, beef, and fish. The judicious use of herbs and spices—such as cinnamon, cumin, saffron, and ginger—enhances the quality of Moroccan food. Fresh vegetables like carrots, potatoes, tomatoes, and onions form the base of many dishes, while lentils, beans, zucchini, eggplant, lettuce, and cucumbers contribute to side dishes and salads. Although not a recipe collection, the book provides educated descriptions of gastronomic marvels, aiming to ignite curiosity and imagination. While restaurants worldwide offer these legendary dishes, the truest enjoyment lies in preparing and savoring them at home.

If you enjoyed this book or found it informative or useful, the author would greatly appreciate your favorable review on Amazon.